Arguments &
& Negotiations

by

Beadrin Pixie Youngdahl Urista

SHIPWRECKT BOOKS PUBLISHING COMPANY

Raising independent publishing to the level of indie music & film

Lost Lake Folk Art
PO Box 20
Lanesboro, MN 55949

IN®
DIE

Cover Design by Shipwreckt Books

Cover Photos by Tom Driscoll

Drawing Page 1 by Pixie Youngdahl

ISBN-10: 098958612X
ISBN-13: 978-0-9895861-2-2

First Printing

I WISH TO DEDICATE this collection of thoughts and musings to every patient who ever allowed me to share in their fear and still found laughter to share; to every nurse, now and in the future, with learned skills, kind intentions and a sense of humor; to my friends and family, far and near, who made it clear they were not finished with me; to all my friends who are writers, Nancy Overcott, Tom Driscoll, David Fingerman and the others who encouraged me from the Minneapolis Writers Workshop. Writers are people who love words and would roll around and bathe in them. And I dedicate this to Tim, who meant it when he promised in sickness and in health; to Jason and Jodi, my kids, who can stop being afraid now, there are more chocolate chip cookies in their futures; to Elizabeth, Andy, Maren and Ellie, the best grand children ever, who are still young enough to hug and kiss their Nanna, even if she is bald.

Lovingly, I dedicate this book to my brother Herve Kermit Youngdahl Jr. (1937 – 2013) who taught me the value of words and ideas.

Contents

I READ ONCE A statement made by a nurse regarding her patients. If I knew the author to credit, I surely would. Instead, I will have to shamelessly borrow the thought:

The only difference between you and me, is you have a diagnosis and I do not, not yet.

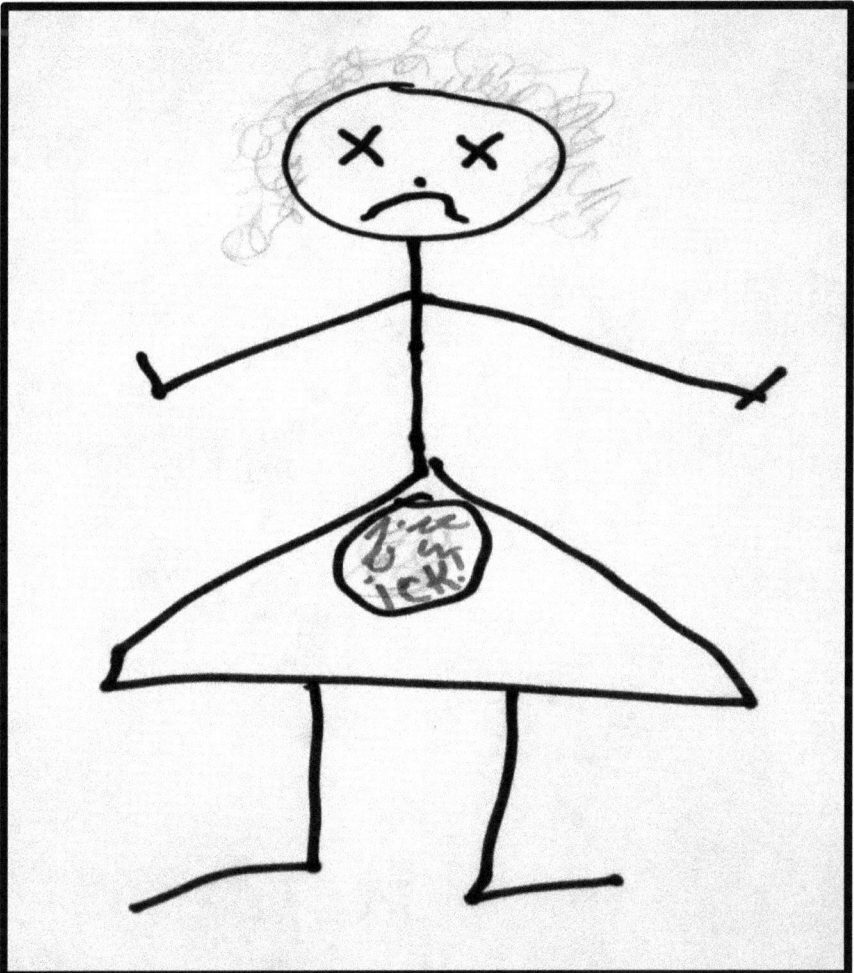

My Turn

THIRTY PLUS YEARS AS a registered nurse had me interacting with cancer in its many forms. I was paid to negotiate with that wily pathology. I ran chemo on people who often suffered more with the cure than the disease, some who finessed their way through it and carried on, and others who did not.

On the brink of my retirement, it is my turn.

Cancer does not roar, it begins with a whisper. Something isn't right. Should it feel like I am sitting on something that oughtn't be there? Hardly dramatic or alarming. Perhaps I am due for a colonoscopy.

The young nurse practitioner listens attentively.

"At your age, I would worry about ovarian cancer."

Well now, wouldn't that be a foolish thing to get tangled up with?

I've done foolish things before but this was the prize.

Pelvic ultrasound, abnormal ovaries. Referral to gynecology and weeks awaiting an appointment. Let this be a sign that it's unlikely to be anything real.

Then comes the real workup. Lab work looking for elevated values on tumor markers. Repeat ultrasound and CT scan. Off to see the gyn-oncologist.

I have worked with oncologists, shared meals, cocktails and great conversation. Now I am in the patient chair. Not a cocktail to be had there, yet where better to serve them?

Information assembled, exam complete and an uncertain verdict. Labs are normal, nothing to be felt on exam, ultrasound and CT are concerning. It could be cancer, but may just be cysts or gremlins in my pelvis.

Laparoscopic hysterectomy is easy surgery. Let's do it and be rid of anything that doesn't belong there. That baby factory went out of business years ago so nothing in there will be missed.

Just prior to surgery, I am told that the doctor expects a simple procedure, in-and-out, home tomorrow, but, (there is always the but), if it is cancer, a full incision will be needed.

It's like Christmas Eve going into the OR, what will I find when I wake up??

Flash forward a few hours spent in a narcotic bliss. I am transferred to a bed in the hospital room and the pain from the full incision is my first indication that mine was not simple surgery. Loved ones are gathered at the foot of my bed, eyes like Hallmark babies looking at me. Ok, I get it.

Jen, my daughter-in-law, is half hidden behind the curtain, either waiting to bolt or to grab Jason, my son, if he tries. Jason is next, first time I've seen him speechless. He admits later that his first thought when the doctor mentioned chemotherapy was, "Shit, we'll have to duct tape her to a gurney to get her in for that!"

Jodi, my daughter, front and center also speechless but big eyed with, "I'm scared and being brave," written all over her.

Kate, a friend and nearly adopted daughter, the first and only to speak and offer the report like the professional she is, repeats precisely what the surgeon had said. Someone needed to step up, explain the situation to me, and it seems it fell to her.

Tim, on the far right, frightened and full of love, silent and watching me.

Cancer.

That's what the doctor said.

My belly hurts too much to rise up and protest the news.

I kick at the foot of the bed, well, shit-fuck. This was not my plan! Give me a minute, I'll figure it out. I need to sleep first. A hit of narcotics and I can start fresh after an escape into slumber. Those who know me well will affirm, my M.O. has always been, "Give me a minute, I'll figure this out."

When daylight comes the doctor is there to repeat what the family said in bits and fragments, or, bits and fragments are what I recall.

It is Stage II Ovarian cancer. He says I am very lucky, most ovarian cancers are not discovered until Stage III or IV, which is why it is so deadly. I was smart to go to the clinic when I did. But I do not feel especially smart or lucky just then.

The cancer was not invading other organs, lymph nodes were negative, but the surgeon washed some errant cells out and, yes, chemotherapy is indicated, sooner rather than later. Only six treatments, they say. Only.

I am *not* a patient! I take care of patients. I am professionally trained to tolerate the whining and crying.

I don't know how to do what they do.

I have never had any interest in learning how to be a patient.

Recovering from surgery didn't take long. They required that I walk in the halls and when the catheter was out the simple act of peeing would win me a ticket home. I peed for the people and walked the halls without supervision.

My nurse chased me down and said, "You aren't supposed to walk without me!" I laughed and told her she had better things to do, that she walked those halls plenty and didn't need a companion. I strolled on and told her, "Don't try to keep up with me. Just carry on!"

I won. Called Tim later and he came for me early in the morning on my second post-op day.

We got home, I sent him on his scheduled hunting trip in Canada, confident I could manage myself. Gege, my sister, insisted that she come to help me so Tim could head north knowing I was not alone.

Gege and I always enjoy time together but she is, in fact, much more frail with health problems than I was with just a gash in my belly. It became a contest to see who was tending to whom. I woke up early on about day six and felt bored and sick of feeling confined. I told her I was getting dressed and we were going to Rochester to a fabric store. She was appalled and tried to talk me out of it.

I rose from the chair and announced that I was going back to bed for a spell and hoped her attitude would improve when I got up. She rolled her eyes and looked a great deal like my mother as I stomped off to my room. When I got up again we compromised on a trip to Winona to run through Target.

Who knew going to Target would feel so liberating? The red and white hundred dollar store seems so enchanting. Cat litter in big bags, paper towels, gee gaws for an already overflowing kitchen, it's all there, calling out to me. My debit card has suffered from lack of use and is happy to see the light.

It felt like I had conquered post-op recovery and was ready for whatever they had in store for what was left in my belly. Ok then, let's do this thing!

Conversations with Me

DARK WINDY RAINY SUNDAY.

Perfect for sewing, knitting and TV watching.

So, Pix, how ya feeling?

My bladder hurts. Not uncommon to get an infection from a catheter in the hospital. Antibiotics assault my tummy. I am learning about the delicate balance between ailments and their cures.

What do you want to journal about?

Don't know. Only know what I don't want to journal about!

No reflections on good health and life.

No inspiration, sentiment or Chicken Soup clichés. If anything interesting is to be said it will be hidden in the ordinary.

My Youthful Oncologist

BACK IN THAT SURREAL world of an oncology office, I am greeted by the perkiest adolescent practicing medicine. I suspect her mom drives her to work. She is clearly skilled and ever so competent but, really, how does a nurse with thirty years experience take advice from someone with still flushed cheeks wearing a size eight skirt?

She makes with all the pleasantries then asks, "So, you are a nurse, you quit smoking for twenty-five years and started again. Why?" (Concerned smile.)

"Because I went to Paris for a week."

"Tsk. Well, I went to Paris for a week and I didn't start smoking."

"You weren't having enough fun. Try again!"

Goody for you, oh perfect one. You're too young to smoke anyway.

She reviewed all the meds she prescribed for side effects and I told her I had some pot I was going to try. Obviously, she has not dabbled there either. "I wish you hadn't told me that. I won't put it in your chart."

I'm not going to mention wine or she'll have me in a treatment program or put me under house arrest for being a senior delinquent. As she matures in her practice, she'll come to see that patients are whole people, not just those frightened things sitting in the chair. I hope I helped her with that lesson.

On a subsequent visit she asked "How are those cigarettes?"

"Great."

She'll learn more effective ways to frame a question, too.

When my youthful oncologist is finished with the teenage, authority-resistant Pixie, she turns me over to the nurses for a poke and five hours of therapeutic poison. Surely the cauldrons are bubbling over with my magic potion. Port-a-cath was placed yesterday and it went well. The Versed-Fentynl IV cocktails are worth the price of the procedure.

My family and loved ones are making it clear they are not finished with me yet, so I guess I must buy the package. Fact is, I'm not done with them either. I'll pull up my big girl pants and do this thing.

The room is large and plush. Huge recliner with heated seat, TV with DVD. The staff is warm, welcoming and well trained in this specialty.

Here we go. One poke into the port on my upper chest and some adjustments on the pump and the first of six rounds of poison starts coursing through my veins.

First is Prednisone and some Benadryl to ward off allergic reactions to the toxic medicine. Then the Taxol, which takes about three hours to run. This is followed by Carboplatin. At the end of the treatment, they actually drain each drop into me, though I know IV bags are always overfilled. I asked why. They reply, the stuff is too hazardous for the bio-medical waste so it's put in me instead. Doing my part to keep Minnesota green!

I am never alone, the book and the knitting I brought remain in my bag. My family hangs out and eats lunch. The staff are in and out frequently. The time does go by easily enough and I feel perfectly fine throughout. See, it's one of the tricks of the trade, fix it so they go home to be sick!

Post-Op Treatment

Friday

I FEEL GREAT! PREDNISONE still acting like cocaine in my system and persuading me that I must be a chemo champ! This is a breeze. I should hire out to do it for others.

Going to the Rushford Clinic for another magic potion. It's a small injection of a fancy and expensive drug to keep my blood counts, specifically white cells, from bottoming out. I can get groceries and run errands while I am in town. I can sing in my car and smile at everyone I see. Still have hair. Over the bladder infection. And healed up from the surgery. Life isn't so difficult after all. The doctor cautioned me that this injection will cause bone pain as the marrow is stimulated to work overtime. I've got Ibuprofen for that. Maybe I'll make a good dinner.

Saturday

THE OOH-AHH BIRD sings with every movement. Did I break my hip? My femur? My thighs would be fine if the drumming with baseball bats could be stopped.

Ibuprofen, hell. I'm back to the post-op Vicodin. And soft whimpering.

Narcotics are the answer, whatever the question.

Sunday

WALKING UNDERWATER. KNOT IN my stomach, no vomiting but I feel like I am hauling road gravel for MnDOT. I won't vomit with the Zofran on board. Can't sleep, can't pace. Couch to bed to chair to couch. Gut full of pills. One pill makes your larger, one pill makes you small.

Tuesday

TWENTY PERCENT IMPROVEMENT IN function, anxiety up seventy-five percent. Pacing. Ativan is the fix.

Thursday

ONE WEEK. THIS SUCKS. The doctor said this treatment was so easy, if I were still working, I would be punching the clock. That could only be true if my full time job was watching *Law and Order* reruns.

If I could sleep, I could tolerate the endless, restless, fatigued days.

Yesterday I swore I wouldn't go forward but I will see how today goes. Making no promises about more.

Who is a stranger to Cancer?

WHY?

WHY DO FOLKS say, "Why me?"

"It's not fair." What is fair? Who better? We are living organisms like leaves on trees, bears and mice. All systems are subject to failure and eventual death.

Everyone is touched by disease and cancer is uncommonly ordinary. To be sure, it is more frightening than a sinus infection or cat allergy but it's all the same to a living organism. Organisms are things to be fixed, to self-heal or to overcome.

I had personal and professional experience with the challenges of this particular pathology. My family is a collective Petri dish for rogue cells to rally. My oldest brother had thyroid cancer at thirty-seven. After surgery, he has gone on without it. My sister had two separate breast cancer surgeries (good thing she had only two breasts or she may have dabbled in yet another), two rounds of chemo and she is now on to other ailments. My other brother had colon cancer last year, rough time of it but carrying on now. The youngest in the family, I waited until all their dust had settled before taking my turn.

My father died at forty-three of pancreatic cancer. He drank too much scotch and vodka so he had all the risk factors. Still, he was too young and I was only five. I remember fragments of him but many of them surround those days at the end.

1957

IT MUST HAVE BEEN a forced march to show-and-tell in kindergarten that would have me standing in front of anyone to say anything on any subject.

Somehow, I was standing there displaying, without narration, a new scarf. The teacher was trying to promote discussion and so, asked me, "Where did you get that pretty scarf?"

"At the hospital." (A girl of few words.)

"Why were you at the hospital?"

"To visit my daddy." (Am I finished yet? Please??)

"Oh? Is your dad sick?"

"Yes, he had Yellow Johnson and then it turned into cancer." My translation of words I'd heard from the adults around me.

I was allowed to go back to my rug at that point. Later, I missed a few days in the spring of that school year to attend his funeral.

* * *

As an adult, and a professional, I found snippets of memory and tried to hold them for him, for my mom, for my siblings, of those days.

Stops

THE INCISION WAS AN unstraight line.

Cross hatched with bloody suture.

A rolling railroad track,

leading from the onset of illness:

"My guts hurt all the damned time,

even when I'm not hung over,"

to a certain terminal end

marked with gladiolas

and organ music.

A meandering route with costly

and painful stops

in hellish places. "After the surgical recovery

we'll try some deep radiation treatments."

Stop

pretending you'll ever be well.

"You see, sir, my husband has been ill

when he is back to work, we can catch up

on the mortgage."

Stop

believing your own lies.

"You can't take dance lessons.

I need you to take care of your sister,

and help with your dad."

Stop

being a child.

"Yes, I can work all the split shifts

my family will manage."

Stop

thinking it will get better.

"Daddy? Why did they cut you?"

Stop

believing in permanence.

A tiny finger traces the wound,

every stop,

memorizing its jagged edges,

waiting for healing

long after the earth consumed

its ragged stops.

Back on the Planet

A FULL WEEK OF recovery time and I am itching to get off the couch, into some real clothes and away from home for a spell. I never knew a trip to Winona could be so exciting. I want to drive my car too fast, play old rock and roll too loud and sing badly with each tune.

First stop, Winona Health for a slightly overdue mammogram. Can't have enough medical procedures. Perhaps I should update my immunizations and maybe schedule a colonoscopy, too!

Next stop, the yarn store to indulge in fabulous wool I had only admired before. Nothing like cancer to support my already refined rationalization skills.

By the time I get home, I confess, I am ready for some couch time and reruns of *Will and Grace*, but my attitude is greatly improved.

Hair Loss

THIS IS THE FIRST thing that cancer patients stress about. It is a daily reminder that something has gone awry. We can't see the disease nor the ravages the chemo can do to kidneys and GI tract. So, we focus on the obvious. I have three wigs, all blonde, scarves of every size, shape and color, knit hats that I sewed but my favorite head covering is a White Sox baseball cap that a friend bought me on a summer day at Comiskey Park in Chicago. The Sox played the Twins that day, so I cheered for both teams.

When I am going out I use a wig or wrap one of my gorgeous scarves around my noggin.

Once I leave the mirror I forget that I'm bald under there. I waltz around with an ignorant confidence and smile at everyone like I always do. I've never been met with any looks of pity, nor any offers to carry this old broad's packages for her!

The hair loss is everywhere. These are things we don't think of until the dry skin on your arms itches so bad you scratch it into bloody rows. Who thinks about nose hair?? Well, it serves a function. It filters air and helps keep nasal mucosa moist. My nostrils make for good sized air tunnels and my nose hurts from the dryness. My eyebrows have fallen out nicely. I always had this Groucho Marx unibrow thing going on and my hairdresser waxes and plucks at every visit. They have fallen out to the perfect light arch I used to pay money for.

Eyelashes, mine are short, blonde and spindly anyway, but there is enough left for a little mascara to grasp onto. I can leave the mirror thinking I look just fine.

Hairless legs and armpits are a pleasant break.

And, we can be grownups, hair is gone in those personal places too. I hadn't seen that little girl hoo-hoo since I was ten. It might be time to take up pole dancing at the Senior Center.

Stretching for Optimism

SOME REALLY COOL THINGS about cancer:

1) I always hated my hair, too fine and no volume despite all the expensive product cluttering my vanity. Perhaps I'll sprout great hair, thick, curly, maybe auburn.

2) Weight loss without hunger. I lost some after the surgery and now drop about six pounds after each treatment and regain three pounds before going back. It might all balance out too, my jeans are feeling better. My real size is an eight but the twelve just feels so good!

3) Won't have to shave my legs for months. Perhaps it's time for a beach vacation.

4) Getting lots of knitting done without any guilt about sitting all damn day.

5) Visits, phone calls, mail from so many good people. I get to find out what I already knew, that my life is full of high quality folks. Having always been drawn to interesting people and, shame on me, intolerant of those who bore me, I now see the final result of selectivity. The best men and women in the world are my friends.

6) I hardly have to do any Thanksgiving cooking. I will stuff the giant bird the neighbors raised for us and just enjoy the family. I could gladly pass the cooking torch onto the next generation and make it a new tradition.

Having said all that, in two more weeks, when I am hating each hour of the long, fatigued days, I will have to remind myself of all this. I know how that will go. I'll look at this list and say, "Pix, you are full of bullshit!"

But, for now . . .

Things to do while dying on the couch from chemo:

1) Watch *Intervention* while drinking wine and smoking. You can wonder if your family would be subject to similar scrutiny, write you treacly letters before sending you off to a plush treatment center and raising your kids while you are gone.

2) Watch the *Food Network* and feel brave about not wanting to eat any of that stuff.

3) Notice the commercials for hair care products and hair removal ads knowing you won't call, even if they will send two for the price of one.

4) Be glad you don't have diabetes or crippling arthritis.

5) Rejoice that this is the only time in your life nobody expects anything from you.

Thanksgiving

SIXTEEN OF MY FAVORITE family members arrive at my door, all bearing food and laughter. It is 60-degrees and sunny.

My four grandkids and two great nephews are wild and screeching all over our five acres.

While food is cooking, the adults gather around the shed with rock and roll music playing, beer and wine pouring and bean bag games in full swing.

Photo ops abound.

My son and daughter are a high contrast in style and personality but have forever been fast friends. To me, even now, there is no symphony in the world lovelier than the sound of my kids laughing together. Growing up, they snitched on each other, lied to cover up for each other, wished they were an only child sometimes but they sure did circle and interrogate one another's choice of spouse! It worked out, they approved after enough shared meals and beer.

Both chose wisely. Both were married 9 weeks apart. Both got into competitive baby making. All the grandkids were born within three years of each other. It's another generation of pals, sharing secrets and mischief. We did well.

My niece gifts me with some pot and a one-hitter pipe. Not the first such gift I have stashed. I now have a nice supply of recreational therapeutics on hand.

I haven't smoked any yet, but when I do, I'll blast some *Rolling Stones* and relive the Sixties like a good Baby Boomer.

If you drive by and see a sign that says Make Love Not War you will know I am feeling ok.

Now, the feast is consumed, the guests are gone, and on Tuesday I go in for labs so they can ok me for another chemo assault. How does passing a test end with a reward like that?

Mid-December

WHAT BETTER TIME TO be sick than winter when there is nothing in particular to go outside for? It is the anniversary of my mother's death twenty-nine years ago. I light a Yahrzeit Candle for her and wonder what she would think of me, bald headed and lazy. Not much probably. She was a quiet Norwegian. She'd have patted my hand and made some coffee. Some days I could still love a cup of coffee with her and of course, some days I still fight with her. Just now, the coffee would be nice.

44

Silent Presence

I HAVE TOLD GEGE that if she ever misses Mom to come to my house because Mom is in my bathroom mirror at six a.m. every day. Dead thirty years now, she seems to have found eternity in my bathroom. I hope she can't see herself, she was a vain thing and I have to say, she looks pretty rough some days.

We meet there and brush our teeth together. She helps me with my makeup, teaching me that make up doesn't help all that much anymore.

At bath time, she returns but averts her eyes in a gesture of modesty, a value she treasured and tried to instill.

She remains silent on the things I would finally like to know. Should this be a surprise? She said little when she had form.

Nonetheless, I inquire on those curious days.

"When you were thirty-seven and got the news that baby number four was coming, how despondent were you in the dark hours when Dad was out partying and you were overwhelmed with the first three?"

"Did you really like eating turkey necks or was that a ritual of self loathing on Thanksgiving?"

"When you didn't sleep at night but sat in the dark with the glow of your cigarette marking your presence at the table, what demons held you there?"

"Don't you think it is safe now to tell me about the cousin who was pregnant out of wedlock and 'went away' for a year? That infant would be retired by now. It is not your shame to bear."

"Those ankle strap shoes of yours that I saw in an old black and white photo. Did you dance in them? Ever? Enough?"

"When Dad died, so young, did you punish yourself for all the times you'd wished it so? Did you forgive yourself for that common wifely curse?"

"Did you ever want to bail out on the entire project?"

"Ok, so you never told secrets but if you did, with whom would you have shared them?"

"When my kids find me in their mirrors, what will they ask of me?"

She remains mute. She'll be back tomorrow, no doubt. If sainthood were mine to bestow, or I thought she desired it, I would withhold it until she 'fessed up, answered me. But then, who needs a saint looking over their personal routines?

In the week after treatment my anxiety becomes more acute than the physical misery. I am fatigued but cannot sleep. My restless legs syndrome, chronic for decades but well-handled with medication, finds a path to befriend the anxiety. They party all day at my expense. I pace. I take pills. I lie down, I get up, I pace. I wish to be put into a medical coma. Unlikely my oncologist will go for that, huh?

It passes in a week. I am so relieved that I choose not to recall it while I groove on being able to go about my regular business. Then comes the day for another treatment, my dog barks in the yard and I jump in my chair. Anxiety is moving in again.

Christmas

I AM A JEW by choice, converted some years ago. However, we still celebrate the traditions of a cultural holiday. This is the first year in forty-one that I have not been with my kids. They are all together, with my sister's family, at my daughters. I am on the couch at home. Merry Merry and Ho Ho Ho, however it lights your candles.

Haven't we all had dreams that were oddly present? Christmas Eve I could not sleep, aching and anxious and so, so tired. Were I more inclined to crying, I'd have been wailing from frustration.

I drifted in and out and found myself back in NE Minneapolis in the home of my junior high best friend and more importantly, her dear mother, my adolescent savior, Alvina. Let me introduce you:

In seventh grade my new junior high friend, Dianne, took me to her house. Heat and the scent of cinnamon assaulted upon entering the back door. We were in Alvina's kitchen.

"Come in and sit down! You have to eat some rolls. I sure don't need them. I'm getting so heavy! I'm so glad Dianne finally brought you home, but I look a mess." She ran her hands through beauty shop hair, probably one day shy of another shampoo and set.

Beauty shop appointments, the great indulgence of the working class in the Sixties. Alvina's ever-present anxiety would grow in the forty-eight hours preceding her appointment until Dianne and I eventually took to setting her hair for her on brush rollers with harsh plastic pins that left dents in her scalp if we fixed them in place especially well.

"I bet your mother isn't heavy," she asked regularly over the years. "Don't I look too heavy?"

She punctuated the question by lifting her stomach with an inward breath, her work-weary hands pressing at its center, offering us a sideways view. No response expected. As the soft folds regained their position she reinforced them with a warm caramel bun, sticky, sweet, billowing with calories and love.

I have her recipe, written in her own hand and style, misspelled, no discernible order, composed entirely of run-on sentences, just the way she spoke. The recipe begins with, "Melt some ole in a pan," and becomes less specific after that. I've tried to follow it, to create the smell and taste and sugary mess of Alvina's caramel buns.

The result is always melancholy. I have the directions but am somehow inadequate to the task. I want to decipher the code within, "Scald milk until hot and add flour until the dough is just right."

Secrets and magic that from my oven become, well, just bread.

I grew up to be a nurse. Dianne married boring men and our lives took different paths. But Alvina, from the first bologna sandwich through all the lard fried hamburgers and eggs fried in bacon grease after sleepovers, fed me love and acceptance with a running apology for all she could not forgive in herself. Her apologies were wasted on me, I thought she was flawless.

She became a patient in the clinic where I worked and I would hold her age spotted hand when she had to have labs drawn. She always dressed up for her clinic visits and I wondered who was setting her hair.

One morning I came to work and the doctor I worked with called me to his office and closed the door. "I got called last night," he said, "Alvina died."

So there she is again on Christmas Eve. I was taking care of my grandkids, her grandkids, all the noise and madness that implies. Alvina told me, "you have to sleep now, just sleep."

I argued that I had all these kids to watch and she promised she would tend to them and would sit right there until I was good and asleep. And she did.

I slept under Alvina's simple, always tender watch. Such things are silly of course, but I'm pretty sure I felt her touch my cheek.

There are things we carry from those junior high halls. Modern math, history, first loves, and the last vestiges of innocence.

Lucky are the adolescents, discovering bad skin and finding their feet too big, their hair too fine, their clothes too ugly, to find a surrogate parent, a special teacher, that becomes as lasting as the stone and brick buildings that shelter them when they are twelve years old.

On Christmas morning, I wake up to an email with videos and photos from my family's celebration, each sending me a greeting. I watch the kids open gifts I sent them.

It makes up for the quiet evening we had. They will come down for New Year's when I will surely be in a more festive state of mind.

A New Year

I AM LIKE A hibernating bear. Not much to do but catch up on old movies anyway. The spring is always our reward and none better than this year, when I am healthy and hauling rocks to place around the gardens. This year I want to teach myself how to build stone walls for my climbing plants. Tim will shudder at the idea but will become engaged when I start digging and stacking. My ideas have typically morphed into his projects. I'm the idea person, he does the heavy lifting.

Back to the Clinic

I'M FINE. I'LL DO it. They haven't killed me yet. As I approach the end of this journey I am surprised that I have come this far. I never expected I wouldn't survive, just that I might buck and quit, like high school.

Ok, my family dragged me every time and gentled me through the recovery. Tim has become a nurse, cook, housekeeper and overall Domestic God. He has put himself at some risk however. I know now he can do laundry and make a bed!

Musings

WOULDN'T ONE EXPECT, IN the wee small hours, some grand wisdom about life might arrive?

Not for me. I work through the same musings I have pondered forever when I am handling gorgeous yarn, completing a quilt project to give to a friend, writing a phrase or two that sound just right.

I have considered the nursing time I spent on the other side of this big chair. I hope I was half the nurse to my patients as I have had so far in this experience. I wish now I could thank each of my patients for the lessons they taught me, when I thought I was the learned one.

Thanks to Mercedes, ovarian cancer, whose husband told her he was sick and tired of her being sick and tired. Mercedes drove herself to and from each harsh treatment. She came in for a treatment once so sick that I took her to the hospital in my car and tucked her into bed there. No husband to be found.

Thanks to Kathy, with a breast tumor at age twenty-eight, three small boys, a now and then boyfriend and a sickly father, her only support. The boys would come with her for her treatments and dash up and down the halls of the clinic. She left this world with those three orphans having very little to hold on to.

Thanks to Clarence with his big voice, big smile and gastric cancer. He continued to hunt deer, dragging them through the woods until internal bleeding landed him in the hospital.

Thanks to the frail ones and the hearty ones. All were a blessing. I have learned this: folks with cancer have their priorities right. No complaints about elbow pain, teeth itching or splitting fingernails.

They treasure the good days, as I do. They taught me about grace and good humor. May their memories be forever blessed.

Getting by with a Little Help from My Friends

I HAVE LONG KNOWN that my life is chock full of high quality people. And now, there is a whole parade of them calling me, emailing me, sending me gifts, bringing me gifts, visiting with me, making me laugh. That's the best part, the laughter.

I am drawn to folks who are witty and interesting. My collection of friends has developed over the years and now surrounds me, all sparkly and colorful. I was never thinking, I'd better save this or this friend for when I get cancer, but here they are.

A friend from St. Paul drove down with lunch for me, books, hand knitted socks and great conversation. The best friends one could ever find in the neighborhood have come by with homemade soup. They are comfortable visiting while I lie on the couch in my robe. My Rabbi and friends from Temple call, then come by with soup, flowers and much to discuss. Ideas make for the best conversation. My elite, i.e. small, writers group friends come by too, email, and don't mind one bit that I am bald. They inspire me to write, to let the chemo kill that internal editor and get words on a page again. My dear friend in Williamsburg, Virginia sends encouraging emails and a card after each treatment. She meets me, laden with gifts, for a treatment in mid-December. Our daughters join us and the five hours we spend together are filled with warmth and really good food.

Friends who arrived from Russia about thirty years ago make a visit to Rochester and we spend an afternoon cooking, eating and catching up. I hear from friends on *Facebook* that have been absent from my life for twenty years or more but renew all my warm memories of time we shared. Gifts of flowers and wine come by mail and Fed-Ex.

I hope never to have to return the favors under the same circumstance, but I surely will. Minus the illness, I plan to reciprocate all the love and kindness. Perhaps one huge party this summer. Stay tuned neighbors, it could get boisterous over here.

Siblings

AFTER MY DAD DIED, Mom worked split shifts as a waitress as well as helping out at the corner store across the street. My siblings took turns watching over me. Each offered a different experience.

Gege was a young teen and took me with her on dates and dragged me to church events, which she loved. Always a failed experiment.

At church, I would hide beneath tables or cling to her legs waiting to get out of that place. Going on dates was a better idea. Once, riding in a car with other teens, she told me we were in St Paul. Outrageous! Minneapolis residents have no reason to cross the river. I thought I'd been kidnapped and threatened to tell Mom.

Orrin had a different style. He would leave me alone, offering to bring back a candy bar, which he would, five minutes before mom got home.

Kerm offered adventures no other kid was able to enjoy in our working class neighborhood. He was an intellectual, or as I thought, just odd.

Fluent in German and French, in the early Sixties Kerm would take me to browse musty old book stores while he hunted for literature written in the original languages. Together, we made long visits to dark and mysterious coffee shops on the U of M campus.

There would be bongo players accompanying poets reading. Kerm would buy me espresso while reading or writing.

I loved being with him. Who knows, I may have seen Bob Dylan on one of those crude stages. Kerm introduced me to jazz before rock-and-roll captured my attention, and to classical music on 33 rpm records in his apartment.

My forever image of Kerm is that of a very tall, lanky man, cigarette glowing, books and yellow legal pads, his voice crooning along with Sara Vaughn on *Lullaby of Birdland*.

In the past year, Kerm's health has declined severely. While I sat at his side in the ICU, sure it would be his last visit there, to calm both our fears I asked him to sing to me. He did. It was priceless. We both survived that episode to share conversations about music, books and movies yet again.

He is in a nursing home now, but still retains that gorgeous rich baritone voice. I have often wanted to record it. I told my sister how comforting his voice is to me and she got one of her big sister expressions and replied, "It is our dad's voice." That explains it.

Gege is as concerned and attentive as she has been since the day I was born. We have never been more than a phone call from each other's reach and are still 'the first call' when anything hilarious or troublesome occurs. We raised our kids together, like barn cats. Any kid needing a hug or a scolding would receive it from the first mom at hand. It's good to keep kids confused about their parentage so more love can be passed around. She is not well either now, but still concerns herself about me. She needn't, but I can't stop her. It's her job.

My brothers, being older than Gege and I, were not so present during those busy years of family. Kerm being fourteen years older than me, and Orrin, ten years my senior, were mostly living out of town during my rebellious years when no adult in the family was eager to challenge me.

Orrin lives in Mississippi, retired from a career in the Marine Corps. Much of his life was spent far from home, including Japan, Vietnam twice and all the home years in the south.

He represents for me an entire generation of young men sent to the jungle to return home again with an eerie and too often destructive silence about the experience. There is a familiarity for most all Baby Boomers about these men. I am grateful that his scars didn't lead him in the too common path of drugs, mental illness and homelessness. I grieve for those who survived the war only to come home to a long hell.

A Little Christmas Larceny

FOR ALL THE LITTLE sisters of that war, I offer the following anecdote:

A Marine Corps issue green duffle bag with its wrinkled and dull colored contents spread wildly around the floor announced that my brother was home on leave. Cigarette debris, already an abundant feature in the house, increased. My mother's voice took on a certain lightness. Her boy was home. To her, all his mess and chaos were as sweet as baby powder on her hands.

An aluminum foil tree with a rotating colored light gave a ballroom effect to the scene: red, yellow, blue, green, again and again. Under the tree, for the first time in his life, my brother had placed gifts for the family. Home after his first tour in Japan, he must have had a mitt full of payday cash on his way to the airport and an overwhelming moment of charity in his heart on his way home for the holiday.

At ten years of age a girl will inventory the Christmas booty daily. My package-shaking skill developed to a high level. Orrin had even wrapped the gifts, or at least he asked a friendly Japanese clerk, one no doubt enchanted by his woeful blue eyes, to wrap them.

The packages were brilliant with color and shine despite their long journey home, boxer shorts and tee shirts pressed all round them.

There was a red one for Mom. For Gege, a square box wrapped in a riot of pine trees on gold background. Just a gesture at shaking stirred a musical response from within.

For Kerm and his wife, a gift wrapped in foil that reflected the primary colors from the spinning light above.

But there was no package for me.

I was not without hope. I looked around and through the packages over and over. I decided it must be an error. I went to Orrin's room and found him smoking a cigarette and listening to county music on a small, black transistor radio. I flat out asked him why my gift was not under the tree. He turned down the radio to accept my query then turned it back up and said, "Why would I get you anything?"

It was clear a new approach was called for. "Did you get me a puppy? Is that why it isn't under the tree?"

"No, I told you. I'm not getting you anything."

In the days leading up to Christmas Eve, I checked regularly for the gift, sure he was teasing me. He would watch me crawl about on my knees with my skinny behind in the air, rearranging and counting packages. The ones that were there held little interest for me anymore. I needed the one that was not there.

"If it's not a puppy, is it a kitten? Did you get me a bike?"

He held his ground, smoked the cigarettes he'd purchased at discount on the military base and brought home in cases for the family. He listened to that little black radio, the technological miracle of the early sixties.

Christmas Eve arrived and I generously gave him yet another chance to slip a bit of magic under the tree. It didn't happen.

Before we sat down to dinner I made a bold move. "If you forgot to shop for me, can I have the radio you brought home?"

"No, you can't. So there, Merry Christmas."

I knew the Marine Corps had cost him some pounds and that his posture was different now, but despite the stubbornness about this gift, he showed no evidence that Corps made him mean. Since he was home, he'd taken me for a malted at the corner dairy store and teased and smiled at me just like before.

It was Christmas though. Mom was beaming as she brought bowls and platters to the table. And I decided I was mad.

I went to his room and found the little black radio. I turned it on quietly and rolled the dial on the side to find a rock and roll station. I wasn't listening to country music for the rest of my life! I shut it off and carried it to my room. The small bedside stand had a drawer for all my valuable treasures, shiny rocks and hair clips mostly. I pulled the drawer out and slipped the radio behind it, replaced the drawer just slightly ajar to accommodate the stash behind.

A smug and satisfied little girl presented herself at that holiday table and smiled sweetly at the soldier brother across from her.

Aunts and uncles and neighbors and friends filled the evening. My brother went upstairs from time to time and became more irritable as the evening wore on. It was late when we settled to open the gifts and I was allowed to distribute them, knowing each and every one from my days of counting and stacking.

Orrin stood by the space heater and accepted thanks and praise from everyone for the gifts he had chosen. Perfume for Mom. An electric percolator for Kerm and Lil. A lacquered jewelry box with a dancing ballerina for Gege. Being the youngest there was no shortage of little girl gifts for me to open and in the litter of paper and ribbon I almost forgot about the gift I didn't get and the Grinch-like action I had taken.

Orrin stood in a sullen posture. As I swept past him with a new game to set up he grumbled, "Hey, if you ever find that transistor radio, it was supposed to be your Christmas gift."

Not old enough to steal and lie at the same time, I threw my arms around his neck in the hug I had been so wanting to give him and squealed, "I know where it is!"

I ran up to my hidey hole and returned with the radio to show the family. It played only rock and roll tunes ever after.

Now my brothers both call before every treatment and a week later to follow up. Perhaps we all see that there will not always be the four Youngdahl kids, and it seems things could change sooner rather than later. Every phone call now ends with, "I love you." Words rarely heard from big brothers before our Golden Years. It means a great deal to me to hear their voices.

The value of the people who have known us forever cannot be underestimated. My siblings are an odd collection of style and personality but they are mine, beginning to end.

Til' Death Do Us Part

HOW CAN THOSE DEWY eyed brides and grooms know what they are promising? They just want to clutch one another until forever. None of us knows of forever.

Neither Tim nor I have suffered great illness. Through flu (always introduced from our school age kids, little vectors) and back pain, colds, minor surgeries, burns, lacerations and bouts of melancholy, we sympathize and roll our eyes as life mates will do.

Tim is frightened of all things medical. He would rather build a wing on a hospital single handed than sit in a surgery waiting room. I had hoped to never put him in that place. He was fortunate to become a father when maternity wards had a fathers lounge where anxious men hung out smoking and watching television, waiting for news from the nursing staff. Had he been in the delivery room, the staff would have had trauma to deal with when he hit the floor in a dead faint.

Now he is a caregiver. I see fear in him, as a spouse will, but his actions deny anything but competence and love.

Housework, cooking, errands, tending to the chickens, grocery shopping and periodic kisses on my forehead are his life pattern for now.

We could have simplified things by transferring my care and treatments to Mayo, Rochester being only forty-five miles from current home. But Minneapolis is my home town, and the care I was offered there assured me that all was well. Tim did not hesitate to dismiss any inconvenience in driving one hundred-fifty miles every three weeks.

One treatment day, the roads were snow and ice covered. I threatened to cancel. He wouldn't hear of it. We took his truck. He'd have dragged me on a sled behind a snowmobile if necessary.

He rubs my bald head and smiles. Can he still see the same girl he met in seventh grade?

I have a modest annuity accrued from my working years. I offered him a trip to Africa hunting as a reward. He said, "You don't have to do that."

It's not near enough.

For Better or Worse

ARE YOU STILL HERE?
You were sure to leave me
when the work headed west
or north, or east. I was only
keeping you until then.
After the wedding, when you realized
how long until forever,
you were just too shy to ask me to leave.
I was willing to save you that
but lacked the courage
to ask for travel money,
so I stayed.
During the high speed years, raising kids,

who had time to look across a room

and contemplate the other adult there?

It's a small team,

you and you

against them.

Certainly the dark hours of quiet

when the kids were crashing through the world

like they were the first to discover it.

We both wondered.

But then, bigger questions entered the mix,

LIFE, DEATH, GOD, PENSIONS.

And now, after all these years,

I want to settle in.

You seem to want me here.

You are finally laughing at my jokes.

Your voice on the phone, midday,

is a soothing surprise to me.

Soon, we'll have to admit

this thing is getting serious.

Expensive by the Pound

I AM TOLD THE little subcutaneous injection I receive the day after treatment to keep my white cells adequate to fight off ordinary infections costs about $5,000 each.

For that, it should make me immune to malaria, snake bite and Bubonic Plague. That is just the little shot to minimize the ravages of the main course.

Lucky me, I married a man who was obsessed with security since he was bagging groceries in high school. However, does that make my health and life more valuable than all those millions who work for poor wages and no benefits?

I think not. What treatment would have been offered had I no insurance? Likely, I'd not have presented to the clinic with subtle symptoms and would have landed in an emergency room when I was riddled with misery. Easy then, nothing to be done.

So I am now a Million Dollar Baby. My dad called my sister his Million Dollar Baby and called me his Two Million. (Can we back up to some of my sister's neurosis and insecurity? Another time perhaps.) I'd be proud to tell him he was a prophet. Not sure this was what he had in mind.

To deal with all the small and large inconveniences of this illness and to be destroyed by the bills as well is beyond my ability. People do it every day. I have no answers and clearly our politicians are inadequate to the task.

This I know, the professionals who provide the care do not drive the problem. They suffer it as well. Mostly they just want to do the jobs they were trained to do. All the advances in medicine let them offer more, but at the end of the day, they do what they have always done with the tools available. They look at the profiteers with the same incredulous expression the rest of us do. Then they carry on.

My surgeon was experienced and compassionate. He had great equipment to utilize, but the expensive equipment would stand mute and hopeless without his skill.

The nurses have electronics galore to aid in their assessments, but they do not replace nursing judgment and instinct to anticipate problems. No electronic miracle can replace laughter as medicine or a gentle voice at the bedside.

Where does all the money go? Big-pharma, medical suppliers, for-profit insurance companies, marketing, and of course, the machine that goes cha-ching.

White Flag Time

IN THE LOBBY OF the Cancer Center gather aged people pushed in wheelchairs by loving daughters, sons or equally ancient spouses. I sit there hoping my scarf wrap is still straight on my head and ponder. How do they tolerate this? Is it their choice to fight the fight or is it the well intended but maybe misplaced concern about family?

Chemotherapy is still fairly crude. It means to target those cells with the black hats but wipes out useful white hat cells as well. If my vital organs were already compromised by age and other pesky chronic illness, I'm not sure I would risk them.

Sometimes we need to ask, "What am I buying?" It's a unique feature of health care. We buy without asking about the price or value. If I bought a car, (the cost of my care could surely have put a shiny new one in the garage!) I would know the price and what to expect. We don't buy clothing without cost and value comparison. If at this time, I was told that treatment might or might not be successful, more information would be in order.

There are thinking people who have a fierce belief in preserving life at all costs. I am not one of those. Whether it is my front row seat to disease and end of life as a nurse or simply my Norwegian practicality, I want value. I have a living will with narrative remarks around all the margins. The bottom line is, when I cannot engage in meaningful conversation, laugh and interact with others, stop the parade and bring in the clowns.

At Last

THE FINAL TREATMENT FEELS right for a party. The course of each one followed the same routine, only the misery and anxiety perhaps lasted a day or so longer each time, or perhaps my patience became diminished, so it felt longer.

Little Dr. Perky comes in prior to the nurses to congratulate me and talk about follow up schedules. Follow up on what? The parts that were bad are all gone, my tumor markers were always normal, there should be nothing to scan, x-ray or draw labs for. I want this behind me and resist the idea of carrying on a relationship with the whole ordeal.

But, I am an obedient patient and schedule an appointment in three months.

I just want to grow hair now.

Tim and Jodi and I go to lunch at *Jax* in northeast Minneapolis when my treatment is finally over. *Jax* has long been our family's favorite celebration restaurant, and the end of chemo sure feels like something to celebrate.

One week later, the port comes out. I am appliance free.

Cancer looks better in the rear view mirror.

Carrying On

IT HAS BEEN THREE weeks and one day since my last dose of toxic waste. Where is my hair, huh? I accepted losing it with some patience and good humor, but now that I am done, shouldn't hair follicles respond? Come on! Its winter and my head is cold!

I am volunteering three days a week and feeling alive and full of capability. Why is my hair lazy?

My kids and grandkids are coming tonight. I have missed them. I want show them that

Nanna does not have to lie about on the couch forever. Maren had a birthday. I am making chocolate cake with chocolate frosting, as she requested. By the way, this is not a box cake, flour sugar and all the rest mixed from my stash in the cabinets.

I will grow hair and not be such a concern to them again sometime soon.

Spring: Myth or Promise?

I'VE DONE SIXTY PLUS Minnesota winters and experience tells me, they always go away. Now, in this post St. Paddy's day snow and ice, I will go on faith.

Spring will arrive and I will examine every plant for signs of life. I will speak gently, coax and make promises about weeding and watering that I'm not sure I'll keep.

My plants know me, they have good fertile ground, sixty feet of buffalo crap to nestle through, and an adoring but lazy gardener to praise their beauty. They forgive me for my neglect and live for my worship.

I intend to be hauling rock from the creek bed to frame them and hope to try my hand at building a stone wall. Tim winces when I suggest such projects because forty years has taught him that my ideas are his labor. Won't a little stone wall be cool though? Sure it will.

I'll sit on the patio he built, with the metal trellis around and overhead, also his design and handiwork, sipping wine and singing to the grape vines. Maybe I can take up wine making as well. What are Minnesotans if not ever-hopeful as spring draws near?

Summer will bring evening fires with rock and roll music blasting from the stereo in the shed, fireworks while the kids chase fireflies, friends and family chatting until well after dark.

These things are promised by the calendar, if not by the current weather conditions. I will be here to realize all of them.

On Task Again

MY SICK DAYS ARE over, blessedly. I had my four grandkids here for spring break when an early morning call came that Gege was in the ICU after falling at home from weakness exacerbated by vomiting and diarrhea. Wait, it gets better. Her daughter, my niece Jen, had a hip replacement at the tender age of forty-one and was staying with Gege for her recovery when the 911 call needed to be made.

I ran from the house and dashed to the Twin Cities to tend to Jen's post-op needs before heading to the hospital where specialists galore prodded Gege for a diagnosis. They had several theories, none definitive. Bottom line, Gege is a train wreck and each crisis adds another bead to her string of ailments that cannot be fixed.

Just after I remarked, "Being the youngest child was cool until all the older children started to crash and burn," the call came that Kerm had passed away at the nursing home. His death was no surprise. He has been ill for a few years with no magic in sight. Still, he is gone.

I will so miss his voice on the phone. I will miss our conversations about music, movies and politics. I am grateful that we spoke just two days before his death when he called to suggest a movie on *Turner Classics* that evening. Most importantly, our conversation ended with me saying, "I love you," and his response, "I love you too, little sis." His voice, always soothing to me, was my father's voice.

His memory will be always, a blessing to me.

Singin' in the Rain

IF I COULD SING or dance, I'd be out there with Gene Kelly and Donald O'Connor, singing, "Good Mornin', good mornin'!" However, I'd surely fracture something in the effort.

When I sing in my car I have perfect pitch and can wail with the best of 'em, Bonnie Raitt, Carole King, Elvis. I lose that skill, however, when I leave the car so it doesn't hold much promise for my future.

If I could paint, I would have a canvas as big as the side of a barn and oil paints, all bold colors. Sadly, my stick people are the peak of my art career.

I will write, as I always have. Writers observe. Writers notice gestures, a lone wrinkle on a shirt, speech patterns, facial expressions and anything that does not fit exactly. Writers love words. To a writer, words have taste and smell and texture.

Writers write to see what they are thinking. They collect images and faces, assemble them into a whole with pen and paper. The words writers choose and utilize, the ideas they express, are often a surprise to them until they read a phrase or paragraph from their own hand and find clarity.

Sometimes writers don't write. So they writhe around in pain instead. I have written more about not being able to write than any other topic. There are poems to be written, but I don't know the words yet.

Writers notice things, even things that don't belong. I noticed, went to the doctor. Noticing has made all the difference.

Stratum

IT IS IMPERATIVE TO GO,

sometime

where the earth curves

to know,

it doesn't end at 5 p.m.

or the county line

or September 11.

Follow that edge

the prairie

the sea.

Seek the line

where the sky curtains down

and makes promises

or tells lies

to its horizontal mate.

* * *

We all look at that horizon and create a fiction about its meaning. Reaching the horizon just means moving forward to the next.

We are all in the business of following horizons. Meet yours, I will meet mine.

About the Author

BEADRIN PIXIE YOUNGDAHL URISTA, a retired R.N. living a quiet life in rural southeast Minnesota, still has deep roots in her home town, Minneapolis. She worked in nursing for thirty-plus years to support her passion for writing, knitting, quilting and now, spoiling her four grandchildren. Nursing taught her much about life, which flavors all the rest.

& Remember.

No matter your skill as an author, Lost Lake Folk Art will enable you to tell your story. We can help you with the writing if required through ghost, surrogate, project writing and complete editorial services. Your life, your farm, your family history or town history, your high school, senior class trip, championship season, the company you built or the one you quit, your first job, first love, honeymoon, your golden years, whatever it might be, it is never too late to capture those memories for others to treasure. Everyone has a story to tell. Let us help you tell yours.

Find more information at

contact@shipwrecktbooks.com

www.shipwrecktbooks.com

P.O. Box 20, Lanesboro, MN 55949

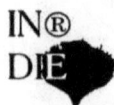

IN®
DIE